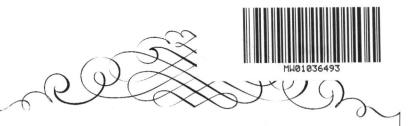
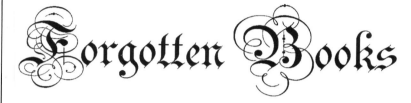
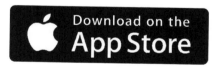
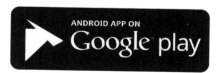

ISBN 978-1-330-30330-6
PIBN 10019939

This book is a reproduction of an important historical work. Forgotten Books uses
state-of-the-art technology to digitally reconstruct the work, preserving the original format
whilst repairing imperfections present in the aged copy. In rare cases, an imperfection in
the original, such as a blemish or missing page, may be replicated in our edition. We do,
however, repair the vast majority of imperfections successfully; any imperfections that
remain are intentionally left to preserve the state of such historical works.

1 MONTH OF
FREE
READING

at
www.ForgottenBooks.com

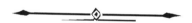

By purchasing this book you are eligible for one month membership to ForgottenBooks.com, giving you unlimited access to our entire collection of over 700,000 titles via our web site and mobile apps.

To claim your free month visit:
www.forgottenbooks.com/free19939

English
Français
Deutsche
Italiano
Español
Português

www.forgottenbooks.com

Mythology Photography **Fiction**
Fishing Christianity **Art** Cooking
Essays Buddhism Freemasonry
Medicine **Biology** Music **Ancient**
Egypt Evolution Carpentry Physics
Dance Geology **Mathematics** Fitness
Shakespeare **Folklore** Yoga Marketing
Confidence Immortality Biographies
Poetry **Psychology** Witchcraft
Electronics Chemistry History **Law**
Accounting **Philosophy** Anthropology
Alchemy Drama Quantum Mechanics
Atheism Sexual Health **Ancient History**
Entrepreneurship Languages Sport
Paleontology Needlework Islam
Metaphysics Investment Archaeology
Parenting Statistics Criminology
Motivational

The Pathology of Dental Infections and Its Relation to General Diseases

WESTON A. PRICE, D.D.S., D.Sc.
CLEVELAND, OHIO
Director of the Research Institute of the National
Dental Association

Annual Meeting
Canadian Oral Prophylactic Association

INDEX

TORONTO
1916

Aims and Objects of the Canadian Oral Prophylactic Association

IN the year 1905 a committee of dentists of Toronto was formed to communicate with the manufacturers of the tooth preparations then on the market to ascertain the composition of each, because they believed that a dentist should not recommend any preparation of which he did not know the ingredients.

Finding there was no satisfaction to be obtained in this direction as to the formulæ of these preparations, arrangements were made to have them chemically analyzed, thus ascertaining that in most of the samples were ingredients which should not exist in an ideal mouth preparation.

The Canadian Oral Prophylactic Association was then organized to have manufactured preparations which should contain nothing which was not beneficial.

After much consideration and consultation a paste was manufactured under the registered name "Hutax" (meaning mouth health). Later a powder was placed on the market, and last a tooth brush.

These articles are the result of frequent consultations with many of the leading practitioners, not only in Toronto, but of the Dominion of Canada and the United States.

The shareholders of the Canadian Oral Prophylactic Association originally subscribed $5.00 each for "the good of the cause," and the charter of incorporation provides that the profits are to be expended for educational and philanthropic purposes, such as (a) bringing prominently before the public important information, which the dentist has, as to the influence of conditions of the mouth on the general health. (b) Care of the teeth of the poor. (c) Assisting the indigent in the profession of dentistry. Thus no director or shareholder receives directly or indirectly any dividends or other remuneration.

Every dentist may recommend "Hutax" preparations with a confident consciousness that there is nothing better on the market, and that the profits will be utilized for the good of the profession and of humanity.

The Pathology of Dental Infections and Its Relation to General Diseases ·

WESTON A. PRICE, D.D.S., D.Sc., Cleveland, Ohio.

Delivered before the Annual Meeting of the Canadian Oral Prophylactic
Association and their guests, the Academy of Medicine,
Toronto, February 14, 1916.

Mr. President,—I want to assure you that I come with a very deep sense of my inability to-night to live up to the standard and desire and hope that has been thrown out by Dr. McDonagh. I think it is a very unfair handicap to put upon a man to make such extravagant statements which of all men I certainly cannot live up to.

It is, however, a very great pleasure to be here, and I come with a mingled feeling of joy that I am privileged to come back to Toronto and be with you again, and feelings of helplessness akin almost to discouragement when I realize the responsibility that is being thrust upon the dental profession to-day, and the utter inadequacy of the dental profession to meet that responsibility. One week ago this evening we had in Cleveland the opening of the Research Institute of the National Dental Association, and had as one of our speakers Dr. Charles Mayo, of Rochester, Minnesota. That splendid orator and magnificent physician and surgeon reviewed to us in detail the development of modern science as it relates to the healing arts. He reminded us of the splendid contributions of the Chinese, of those great contributions of the Greeks, and finally came down to the present decades and reminded us how one after another the great scourges, the great besoms of death, had been taken from the earth by medical science, and then as his climax, said the great mass of people to-day would not die of one of those plagues, they would die of a simple infection, that 90 out of every 100 probably would die because of some simple infection, the result of a focal infection, which focus itself would give them no trouble. He then referred to the fact that 90 per cent. of the lesions, of the focal infections, are above the collar, and of those above the collar which would include the tonsils, the antrum, the nasal passages and sinuses, that for the largest part come from dental infections, oral infections, and then accepted the challenge of the dental profession that they are going to take that responsibility. Are you going to do it, brothers? Recently I have been corresponding with the deans of the universities and the dental colleges of the country, with the editors of our best journals, and advertising in our dental journals to find if we cannot get one dozen, or even one-half dozen, men who are competent to go into the department of research to determine the relation of mouth infections-to systemic infections. How many do you suppose we could find? I am ashamed to let you know. There are a few good men who are doing research work, but we cannot pry them loose from where they are, but alas, the tragedy is we haven't men in the world to-day; we haven't enough to even do one per cent. of the work that is demanded right now in interpreting the relation of mouth infections to systemic infections, and vice versa. Dr. Mayo said last month that at this moment we should have four dentists to every one that exists now in order to look after the interests of humanity. Not only for their own sakes, but for the State's sake. What does that mean? Well, my dear brothers in the profession, it means we must put our shoulders to this wheel. We have a great responsibility as a dental profession, namely, to help interpret the relation of these mouth infections to systemic infections. He also said to me on that occasion, as he did in Boston some weeks ago, we have learned as a medical profession doing research as we are in our institution, that these problems cannot be solved by medical men; they must be solved by men with a dental vision. Where are the men with the dental vision?

Unfortunately, when we try to pick out the men with dental vision, that is all they have got. Oh, the men with the medical and dental vision are the men that are wanted; the man who is big enough to see all the physician sees, and also see what the dentist sees—these seeing both at once are the men we need. I visited a hospital in Chicago not long since, and one of the leading bacteriologists took me through one ward after another and showed me the many cases that were being treated and helped, because they had treated the mouth infections, and then we came to a room, and he said: "There is a great joke in this hospital. We have got to get a new room to store the teeth in. As a matter of fact we are extracting so many teeth in this institution we have really got to get a new place to store them." I said to him, "What proportion of the teeth that are extracted in this hospital are in your judgment related to the other infection that the removal of the teeth did cure or did relieve?" He said, "I have thought of that many times, and I have thought that three or four out of a dozen." The average number of teeth extracted in that hospital under the direction of the medical men, he said, was about twelve, and in his judgment as a bacteriologist not more than three or four of the twelve ever should have been extracted. We are honored, I understand, and I am glad it is so, to have a number of the medical men with us to-night. I don't know what your practice is here, but I do know that I go to cities where the feelings of the medical men sometimes are so extreme as to even demand that every tooth that has a dead pulp is a menace and should be removed, and if it isn't giving trouble it may give trouble.

Now, that is almost as extreme as a physician as perhaps are 70 per cent. of the dental profession, who rather plume themselves and say, "Well, perhaps so and so is not competent to save this root, but I can put a bridge on that will be all right." I say the dental profession are taking the other extreme and are saying, or thinking, and are allowing themselves, perhaps, to be misled—or else they have not informed themselves of the danger— and they are going right ahead and putting dental work on teeth that are already shortening the lives of those patients. I believe and know, just as much as I know I am standing here, that a lot of my dental operations have helped to shorten the lives of patients. I would give a great deal if I had not done some of the work that I have been doing. I believe absolutely that I have put bridges on to teeth that already had an infection, and that were undermining the health of those patients, and I did not suspect it. I have had the privilege of undoing some of that work, and if God will spare me I hope to undo quite a lot more of it. To show you that I have not been a gold crown advocate I may say I have never put a gold crown in any person's mouth forward of the second bicuspid. So you see I have not been a slave to the gold crown habit. I have refrained from devitaliz- ing pulps where I could accomplish the result in some other way, but I have felt I was so skilful that I could attach bridges to teeth that had deep pyorrhea pockets beside them. I thought I was so skilful that the patient was wonderfully fortunate to be in my hands, but I know very well that they would have been better off in the hands of some man entirely unknown to the community, but who with his conservatism was satisfied to practice a great deal less scientific dentistry perhaps, but would use the forceps more frequently than I would. Well, some medical people will say, "That is what I expected, and that tooth should be extracted." That is just as far from the mark as the other statement, for the time has come when we can distinguish the type which is a dangerous type of infection from one which is not. Now, which is the greatest tragedy which has de- veloped in this entire field of research during this last two or three years? I know of none that is so significant and so appalling, because of its subtle- ness, as the abscess. The dental abscess that is causing trouble in the mouth of the patient is, as a rule, not the one that will be causing arthritis or myelitis, or a heart affection, not nearly so as that type of dental abscess that produces no local trouble. Let me repeat: Of the last dozen cases that we have studied and treated for arthritis there has not been a single exception to the fact that the lesions which we relieved and treated improv- ing the patient's condition were giving no local trouble. Why? The very type of infection answers the question. What do I mean by the type of infection? Here we have a rapidly developing abscess with a great deal of inflammation and pus formation. We have not got a simple strep- tococcus infection; we have a stercoremia infection, with some of the ancillary contaminations with it. But when we have a pure streptococcal infection of the type that produces lesions that I referred to, almost in- variably, if not invariably, they give the patient no trouble. Now, this seems like a contradiction, but if that organism produced a very much more severe reaction in the human body it would be a great deal better for the body—if it was worse it would be better. That seems like a strange thing, but what does that mean? If an organism growing in your body starts up some trouble in the body and brings forward the resisting powers of the body a new element is created, a chemical substance that reacts against that organism, and the body politic, our united body, drives it out. We build up a resistance, I say, and we destroy the organism. Why? Because it irritated our bodies. But when it grows within our bodies without producing an irritation the body does not react, and therefore there is no anti-body built up to destroy it, and consequently it lives on and on and the body is almost indifferent to its presence. Here is another strange but rather important apparent contradiction. The lower the virulence of the organism the more subtle it seems to be in producing these grave lesions like the arthrities. The lower the virulence of the organism the less tendency it has to produce a reaction on the body, and the more certain it is to produce those lesions like the arthrities. Now, we will see some reason for that. If we were to go down to a restaurant to-morrow morning, and if you would take along with you several other species besides the human species—let us say a porcupine, a grasshopper and an ant—you all go into the restaurant, and we will assume you are all going to order from the bill of fare. What would be the difference in the meal you would order? As a matter of fact you would all order nearly the same thing. What would it be? It would be largely protein. Why? You have a digestive apparatus that would digest a nice piece of chicken, like we had this evening, and I found my digestive apparatus inside could dissolve that chicken splendidly. Now, the porcupine would not take that. He would select a nice piece of bark, and another of the organisms would select a piece of horn. You could not digest the horn, and you could not digest the bark, so those various forms of life would select the very thing that they could digest. The point I am trying to emphasize is that the only difference between you and every other form of life, including those streptococci, for example, is that your digestive apparatus is just a little different to theirs, and yours changes and theirs changes. They have the property of living on certain tissues of your body, and your body has the power of taking in food, and can select certain of those products for different organs of the body. Let us assume you have taken your piece of chicken. How does that chicken become part of your muscle tissue? You have two different kinds of digestion, and the micro-organism has also. You have two kinds of digestive fluids, one in the stomach, another in the arteries and veins, in the blood stream, a digestive circulation, and the protein you take into your body, as, for example, the piece of chicken, is split up. It does not go into the body as a whole protein; it is divided up as you take an axe and split up the wood into fibres, and afterwards it goes into that other circulation. Then each cell of your body has digestive fluid, and these take the particular pabulum that it wants, just as your body, which is a multiple of cells, and each streptococcus has one digestive fluid outside its body and one inside its body. All living things must do three things; they must eat, they must assimilate, and they must excrete, and you and the·pabulum are precisely alike, as we will see from different viewpoints as we go along. When you take into your body some protein which gets into your circulation, which has not been properly split up in your stomach, what happens? Why, immediately the chemistry of your body is called forward and you build up a new enzyme, a new chemistry, to dissolve or digest that very thing; and the thing that happens is this: If, for example, you have got, we will say, an overdose, you have overeaten, in other words, bananas or eggs or milk, or any kind of food, in so large quantities that some of that protein gets from your stomach through into the circulation without having been properly split up, the blood immediately produces a chemistry that splits up and digests that protein that has gone through, and ever after that if you eat eggs or bananas, or whatever the thing is that has poisoned you, immediately that chemistry is ready and splits up that protein, and that protein when split up in your blood is part poison, and that poison is the thing that $_{is}$ making you sick, and you can't eat those things. When you get typhoid fever, for example, the organism grows in your body, and that is precisely what happens. You react—that organism in your blood has called forth the new chemistry which tears down and splits up those organisms, part of which are poison, and that poison makes you sick. You are walking up and down the country with those organisms in your body; they are incubating in your system, but it is not until your body reacts that you are sick. What does that mean? Simply the time comes when this chemistry is so perfectly developed that immediately the new organisms come into the body the defensive forces rush to the rescue and produce a large amount of this chemistry and destroy that organism.

Now then, what happens when the bacteria of your mouth, for example, get into your blood system? They do not stop there, and consequently a resistance of the body has not been stimulated, but pretty soon your body builds up that chemistry, and immediately it does you' are sensitized to it, and day after day your body is reacting to that very thing to which it is so sensitive. Now, what is the significance of this? Many of you know this, but for those who do not I will call it to your attention. If you were to take a little of the white of an egg and inject it into your circulation to-day—just the ordinary white of egg which your stomach would digest—if you inject it into your blood system circulation to-day it would not do you much harm; it would be in there as a foreign substance, but your body immediately builds up the chemistry to destroy that protein, and in ten or twelve days if you put a little bit more white of egg in it will kill you. Why? You have been sensitized to that white of egg, and even so small a fraction of any of the proteins as sometimes the millionth part of a dram will be enough to sensitize the body so that when the subsequent dose of that gets into the blood system the reaction is most violent on the part of the whole body, because it so rapidly splits up that protein. You all have seen this illustrated, for it is the man that is apparently the strongest that dies with typhoid. Why is that? Because he had to tear down so many of those organisms immediately that his reaction has been stimulated. · So it is the strong men that die of this disease, because nature reacts so violently and so much of the poison is set free. There are scores and scores of people that are going up and down our streets suffering from a poison that is going into their body by absorption of protein from the bacteriological infection of their mouths, and they are sensitized to it; the dental operators know what I speak of so well. You know that if we undertake to scale too many of the teeth the same day they are violently sick. I remember one woman where I simply took care of about one-quarter of the teeth, removing the debris from the teeth, because in that operation we open up the circulation slightly and let in more of these toxine poisons, and I said to her, "This is all we had better do to-day; let us stop now and you telephone me to-morrow and let me know if you have had a reaction," and although that woman had walked to the office and walked away apparently in her normal health, which was much below par, the next day, even with the telephone within arm's length of her bed, she reached to get it to telephone me, as she had promised she would tell me how she felt, and she was so sick she threw herself back on the pillow and said, "What is the use?—he told me I would be sick anyway." She was simply reacting to the toxine, to the protein that was being absorbed from that poison. Now, that is going on in a large degree in so many bodies, and there are probably hundreds and thousands of us that are beginning to die at 40 and 50 years of age because we are over sensitized to those mouth protein poisons.

Now, I will not have time to go very far into that discussion, and I will take the slides at this time and discuss first some of the typical kinds of lesions, and because of the impossibility of covering the ground I should like to limit myself very largely to streptococcus infection. The first slide which we will put on will be one showing the Research Institute of the National Dental Association, a building that has been purchased for the dental profession of the United States, a building which contains something like thirty rooms, and I am glad to say that within six weeks after the call went out to the dental profession for assistance to buy that building one-third of the entire cost of the property was in our hands, either in cash or pledges. It is also significant that these researches that have been going on now for about three years, and which have entailed an expense of something like $75,000, 90 per cent. of that amount has come from the dental profession as voluntary contributions. This building which you see has something like 30 rooms, and has another building at the rear with a splendid auditorium, and we have facilities for taking care of a large amount of research work. I will be glad to furnish anybody who is interested with a more detailed description by mail.

In this picture we have a typical infection of a streptococcus type, producing no general disturbance. This patient was out of business for four years, and for two years of that time was in sanitariums and hospitals. He had symptoms of gall-stone and peptic ulcer, or stomach disturbance of various kinds, and twice was taken to the hospital for operation. On both occasions it was decided not to operate, because it was so uncertain that there were gall-stones present. He had fallen off in weight from 156 pounds to about 120. Twenty years previous to the time of the presentation of the patient he had a boil on his chin, which in all probability was an external fistula to a dead pulp in a tooth. It was not recognized that the pulp in the adjoining lateral was dead. Our examination with the radiogram showed the presence of the abscess. We opened into the right lateral and removed some of the infection and inoculated it, and studied the organism with our various methods, and were able to produce in animals the typical liver infections. By typical I mean corresponding to the infections that we get consecutively with that type and strain of streptococcus. With no other treatment than obliterating the area of infection at the two roots, opening up the canals and thoroughly cleansing, this gentleman gained 25 pounds in twelve weeks, and went back to his business.

He lived in another city, and his physician has written me that he has no doubt but what we did remove the entire cause of this man's trouble. The last time the man called on me he said he worked from seven in the morning till eleven at night, and looked as stout and well as could be. The next slide shows the typical lesions in the animal, and the section of the liver shows a typical focal abscess, which we get with this strain of streptococcal infection. I want you to note that the blood vessel is entirely blocked. The kidney of this animal shows a cloudy swelling, but without an abscess, that is very characteristic of this type of infection. Here we have the picture of a young man who was treated in the clinic of Dr. Hartzell, who is one of our directors of research supported by the Research Institute, and working in the University of Minnesota and in the hospitals. This man had not been without pain for nine months, and could not walk, could not feed himself, could not put on his own collar and could not dress himself. At the time this picture was taken, as you can see, he could put his hands behind his back and up over his head. The next picture shows us the lesion that was found. This man had been in the hospital for nine months, and the treatments given him were doing him no good, and he was turned over to our department. The medical men were not able to satisfactorily find relief for the infection. The area of absorption is shown around the molar. The removal of the dental infection and the making of a vaccine entirely removed the trouble, or sufficiently so that he was dismissed from the hospital in six weeks. He could then run up five flights of stairway in the Donaldson building, one foot above the other, where five weeks before he couldn't put his foot to the floor in the hospital, and no other treatment than the removal of the infection and the vaccine made from this culture. Here we have another case from Dr. Hartzell's clinic. This woman had suffered for three years. You notice the ankles are swollen, and the knees and the hands, and she is very much emaciated. She suffered very great pain, and month after month they were placing on record "present treatments doing patient no good." The next picture shows us the dental infection at the apices of some old roots, and with no other treatment than the removal of these roots and the making of the vaccine the trouble was removed. We do not emphasize the vaccines much. We believe they are helpful in certain cases. In a few weeks this woman was able to stand erect on those knees that had not been straightened for many months. She was dismissed from the hospital and went back to her family of several small children who needed her very much. She has had no recurrence in twelve months. Here is a case from my own practice. We had watched this patient getting worse for fifteen years and we came to the conclusion that some dental trouble was the cause. The next picture shows us the area of infection around the bicuspid. With very little other treatment than the treating and removing of that infection and the imperfectly filled root which I had filled some twenty years before. The radiogram which has done splendid service showed the imperfection, and that woman now has thrown away her crutches. This picture shows a patient that is being carried to my office. The woman could hardly move her head or elevate her hands, but with no other treatment than treating the dental abscesses in that woman's mouth those joints that were so tied up that her knee joint could not be flexed one-eighth of an inch will now swing through quite a large arc, and very soon she will be on her feet. The pain is entirely gone and she has gained a number of pounds in weight. I think she will be walking around by midsummer at the rate she is improving. When that woman was put in the chair she could only move her head half an inch without moving her position on the chair, so rigid were her vertibrae, and now she can turn her head from side to side and look over her shoulder, and that is from the treatment that has taken place since November. I am sorry that I failed to bring the slides showing the infections in that woman's mouth. There were five abscesses all at the apices of teeth that had had dental treatment, some with gold crowns and some with fillings. Only one of the five had a fistula. Every one of those teeth except the one with the fistula gave us a pure culture of the strains of streptococcus, and the one with the fistula gave us a mixed infection. Now, what is the significance of the fact that those teeth did not give trouble? That woman's teeth had been examined in the hospital for nine months, and this condition had been coming on for nine years, and they pronounced her mouth in perfect condition, and when I looked into her mouth without the radiogram I said there is only one tooth indicating an abscess, and that was the one with the fistula, and the tragedy is, as I repeat, that the very conditions that will give these grievous troubles seem to be invariably those which produce no local trouble. It means we can not trust our own methods without having radiograms taken. Then we have here the case of a young man twenty years of age. His mother has been in bed for five years with an arthritis, and he has been suffering considerably with arthritic infection of increasing severity. I want you to note the anterior buccal roots were not filled. You notice the areas of infection. Our method of getting cultures practically in all these cases now is to get the culture from the apex of the root without the extraction of the tooth, before the extraction, in order that we may get a pure culture, believing that we can get the infection more perfectly and safely without extracting the tooth than by extracting. We did that in this case, and out of five in that area we were able to get the pure streptococcal culture of three by aspiration. There was no extraction done and yet he has had his infection apparently entirely relieved. I say that with the emphasis on "apparently." I believe that that young man is in danger of having that infection recur. I doubt very much whether I have ever sterilized the area beyond the apex of a root by any medication that I have ever been able to use—I say thoroughly sterilized. I think we greatly reduce the infection at the apex, but I doubt if we entirely remove the infection. This instrument that we use for aspirating, has a long rubber tube to it and has either glass tubing or copper tubing slipped into a glass tube and aspirate into the tube by sealing the small copper tube into the root of the tooth with wax or cement, preferably with cement, and almost invariably we can get a culture of the infection in the root of the tooth by aspiration, whether or not we can locate the organisms in the root itself. Dr. McDonagh requested me to leave one of these instruments with him and if you are interested he will be pleased to assist you in making one a great deal better than we often see. We find it a most indispensable instrument in connection with the treatment and diagnosis of these conditions.

A great many of the infections of the mouth select out tissues that we had not suspected a few months or years ago, and I will now show you a few slides illustrating that. The one I am presenting is of a woman who is teaching in our public schools and who had to give up her profession on account of losing her voice. There was no apparent cause, but with no other treatment than the removal of an infected and impacted cuspid, and it was due to the infection not the impaction, that young woman had her voice entirely restored. The next slide shows the case of a young woman, now not a very young woman, for she has lost her voice for something like twenty years, or nearly lost it. She called me up on the long distance telephone the day before I came away, telephoning from another city, to show me that she could talk now with her voice, the first time she had talked long distance for a great many years, and her husband says her voice is better now than any time in nearly twenty years. She had no other treatment than the removal of the dental infections. Another important characteristic of a streptococcal infection of this type is that the alveolar bone does not recover normally as appears with other types of infection. Many of our dental men present will recognize this condition shown on this slide. Here we have a first molar, and you will see the area of infection at the apex. This gentleman had suffered from recurring inflammation of the throat and chronic bronchitis that took him to the doctor almost every week. After the infection was removed he has not had a recurrence for two years except a grippe infection, which we could not assume was caused by the old infection. I want you to note this, that the result is that the bone does not restore perfectly. Now, why? We found three months after the extraction of that tooth that we could get strains of that organism from the alveolar bone surrounding the socket by drilling into the bone. I feel very strongly that practically every case of streptococcal infection of this type which is of a very low virulence, will carry that infection for many months in the bone around that socket, and every tooth that has such an infection must have a very thorough curettement to remove that infected bone, and not trust to simply the removal of the tooth for obliterating the infection. That is a thing that we as dentists have not appreciated. Sometimes the infection may be very extensive. Here is the case of a rather beautiful woman who got an infection in the mandible from the central incisors, lower, the result of which was that a necrosis destroyed the entire mandible so that she lost all the teeth from the third molar on one side and the second molar on the other and the mandible from the third molar on one side to the second, on the other. The chin was gone entirely, practically. That was not a streptococcal infection. We do not get much if any pus flow with this type of infection. As a rule those extreme infections do not come from the type of organism that will produce these disturbances. While we are at this I will ask you to note that the stretching pressure on the new forming bone was sufficient to make that chin grow out to almost its normal position. Here is a picture of the same woman as we see her on the street to-day, and again she has got a chin. By having that bone stretched as it was growing about an inch and a half of new bone has been made to grow out of about half an inch of bone that attached those two stumps. She could only take a liquid diet when we started that stretching operation, and now she can eat as large a meal as anybody of as coarse food practically.

There are some types of infection that will be carried in dead teeth for a great many years. The next is the case of a woman whose teeth were giving no trouble at all, but they were discolored. I felt that it was my duty to remove the dead and putrescent pulp. I opened into the dead tooth after demonstrating that it was dead, and that tooth that was giving her no trouble took on an active form of inflammation so severe and rapid that by ten o'clock that night she had a fever of 103, and the next morning when she came to the office her head was all tied up and she had a very high fever and very much prostrated, so much so that she almost had to be carried in and threw herself on the lounge. By that time we had made a sufficient study of the organism to identify it. It was a free baccillus which grows with two expressions. When it does not get oxygen it produces very slight inflammation locally, but by opening up the tooth and letting the air or oxygen in we get an entirely new expression from that same organism, and the opening up of the tooth allows it to take on a new condition of very grave irritation. We asked this woman if she had had any severe illness, and she said seven years previously she had pneumonia. This bacillus very commonly grows along with the organism of pneumonia, and in all probability this tooth had its vitality lowered at the time of the pneumonia and it remained there all these years, and this illustrates how a patient may carry in the body an organism that is ready at a moment's notice to re-infect with a very grave infection, which organism came in at the time when they had some general infection, and that suggests what so many dentists in this room have seen over and over again, an epidemic of abscessing teeth. Now, I find very few physicians have sympathy with that. They do not understand that, but as a matter of fact the men of the dental profession have had the experience of seeing, perhaps, more abscessing teeth in two weeks of one period than they may have seen for six months before or after. What is the trouble? A streptococcal infection is going about, or some other form of infection, and the organism goes through the system and lodges at the apices of the teeth where there is a good culture medium, and immediately that patient is troubled with abscessing teeth, the infection gets to the teeth through the blood stream and causes that epidemic.

VALUE OF VACCINES.

The next slide is particularly interesting because it shows where a third molar was extracted, and under normal conditions the alveolar bone has restored more in six weeks than in some other location it would in six months. This is a streptococcal infection that was producing a chronic irritation of the throat with bronchitis, which cleared up entirely after the removal of this infected tooth. This slide will suggest to us the use of vaccines. Where shall we use vaccines, and how much of them shall we put in them, and what kind of vaccine will we use? We have the extremes of opinion in the dental profession as we have in the medical profession, but my judgment would be and is that vaccines can be beneficially used in very carefully selected cases, but we are liable to place altogether too much confidence in them.   This slide shows a young woman twenty years of age who had a necrosis going on for something like four months which did not subside or respond to local treatment.   She was overwhelmed with an infection, and the making of a vaccine from the contents of this pocket which is shown completely changed the condition. The pus had stopped almost entirely in three or four days and the sinuses were healing up.   Before that time we could inject a solution of medicine into the seat or focus of this necrotic area we had to get at both the lingual and buccal to the third molar, and even the second molar, and with no other treatment this picture was changed completely and the young woman was restored in a very few days to health again.

The next picture shows a gentleman fifty years of age.   A vaccine was made, and the restoratives gave him improvement for something like five weeks and then lost its efficiency entirely.   Now, what is the difference between these cases?   If you have people with lots of resistance and lots of reserve who are suddenly overwhelmed by infection you may bring out nature's hidden strength, as it were, by means of a vaccine and help them to overcome this temporarily overwhelming infection, but with people beyond fifty years of age we must not expect much from vaccine.   The next slide shows one of the tragedies of our modern splendid dental service.   This man was willing to pay for the best dental service that could be got in the world, and he was able to pay for it, and was trying to pay for it, and yet for something like five years he has been compelled to deny himself practically all the privileges of public life because of irritation of the bladder, and during the last twenty years he has been suffering with that trouble.   A bacteriological culture from the urine gave us a typical streptococcal infection.   The radiagram showed this area of infection where the absorption had been going on for years.   We got a very prolific streptococcal infection, and with no further treatment than the treatment of that tooth which the dentist had very securely anchored to the next tooth back of it, with no other treatment than the extraction of that tooth the irritation of the bladder cleared up.   Now, is it not a tragedy that we as dentists will hitch onto a sick old tooth which nature would eliminate if she could?   We will hitch it onto some good healthy tooth and prevent nature from throwing it off, and I have no hesitation in saying that the Cliff Dwellers with their healthy mouths without decay were infinitely better off than our civilization with our boasted dentistry, because we do not know better than to hitch sick teeth onto well teeth.

This slide shows the case of a whole series of infections nearly, starting at first with an acute inflammatory process in her joints, then a heart infection, then a liver disturbance, so much so that they thought she would have to be operated on for gall stones and then peptic ulcer.   Then finally a carbuncle from which her physician thought he took a teacup full of pus, if such were possible, and then when I saw her at one time I think she had probably a hundred boils of various sizes.   Her physician said he did not take any stock in all this bunco about mouth infection, and he didn't think the bad teeth had anything to do with it, and if she didn't want them out she didn't need to.   Now, that to me is a tragedy, that the men of our dental profession cannot have the united co-operation of the medical profession, and I use that as an illustration, and I hope it is a rare one.   I am sorry to say it is not a rare one in our city to find medical men who do not yet recognize the importance of mouth infection.

Now, I wish to differentiate between mouth infections and lesions produced by impacted teeth and the lesions produced by pus under pressure. We were told by Dr. Mayo last Monday evening that pus will produce a typical type and successive chain of expressions of the nervous system; when not under pressure, produces an entirely different type of expression; when under pressure, coming not from pus but from an impacted third molar, we get a re-action on the nervous system that is entirely different, and very often involves a mental disturbance so grave that we will have these people locked up in our sanitariums.   Here we have the case of a young woman who has been in an asylum for two years, part of the time in a plaster of paris jacket because she was so violent.   She had all sorts of hallucinations.   With no other treatment than the removal of the impacted upper third molars and the removal of the remains of the distal root of a second molar that was entirely grown over she was completely relieved so that in two weeks she was dismissed from the asylum as cured, and has been for the last nine months studying grand opera in Boston, putting in five hours a day at her studies and is apparently perfectly well again.   I want to emphasize that the type of expression that comes from an impacted tooth is quite different from the expression that comes from a septic infection, and with no other indication but the deposit as shown in the next slide we will have an acute inflammatory process take place.

I presume one of the greatest contributions that has come from this entire field of research has been made just recently by Dr. Hartzell by showing that even the amount of infection we may have in these spaces will be sufficient to gain entrance directly through the open lymph channels and blood vessels and infect the apices of roots, and a little more deposit produces this amount of inflammation.   This slide shows what I should say is our graveyard of dentistry, the gold crown.   I do not know of any operation that we as a dental profession have made that has produced so much local and general disturbance as the gold crown, because with it we may cover up an infected pulp, and not only that but primarily we may produce an irritation at the gingival margin and by that irritation start an infection that may involve not only the tissues around the tooth but involve the apices and all the periodental tissue, and secondly, all the tissue parts of the body. Very frequently I have slides referred to me such as these, although these were taken from Dr. Black's book, where particularly the medical profession are not interpreting the slides correctly. Here we have a dental abscess for example, which is not a dental abscess, but a nerve foramin.

This slide is put in to show you the proper position of the X-ray tube to get the proper light and shade. If, for example, we have the angle of the rays at right angles to the long axis we will get a lengthening of the root, and if we make the angle of the ray at right angles to the film we will have a shortening of the tooth. The proper position or angle of the rays is at right angles to a plane which is halfway between the long axis of the tooth and the plane of the film as shown in the lower picture, which will always give you the shadow of the tooth the same length as the tooth itself. This slide shows the type of dental lesions that may produce very serious systemic infections without local disturbance, for practically all these cases were not giving local disturbance, and yet they were giving serious systematic disturbance. Here we have the typical abscess with a fistula into the hard palate. Here we have a blind abscess, and of all the types the blind abscess is by far the most dangerous and serious because it produces a type of infection that does not make a local disturbance usually, but does produce serious systemic disturbance.

If we had time I would like to emphasize the difference in a number of organisms in a healthy mouth and an unhealthy mouth. If for example we take the amount of debris from a decaying tooth that would be represented by a milligram, an amount that you could carry on the head of a pin almost, and count the organisms in it you would have all the way from 10,000,000 to 250,000,000 or 500,000,000 organisms in that small quantity, a thing we have not dreamed of, and when you realize that that milligram of material would only be a fraction of the total amount in the mouth we get an idea of the amount of infection we are carrying around with us. Then if we note the different types of mouths and the amount of infection in each we will readily see that an immune mouth with 10,-000,000 and a dirty mouth with primary caries with 500,000,000 organisms we have the answer almost immediately for the decay, the number of organisms being almost in proportion to the decay, and I have here a slide with the columns illustrating this

If we had time to go into study of the pathological aspects, we would find this gingival notch to which I am pointing on the outside of the tooth may have so slight an infection that the gum is only slightly reddened, and yet the blood vessels as shown by Dr. Hartzell will come to within three

or four or five microns of the surface, and all the germs have to do growing in that area is to travel through that four or five microns of distance,
and when you consider that a micron is the 25,000th part of an inch, and
when you realize they have to go less than 1,000th part of an inch to get
directly into the veins you get an idea of what importance it is not to have
the seal broken at that point. The human body is a sealed envelope as
nature intends it to be. If any one of us had an abscess area as large as
a penny on our hand our physician would be very careful to have it covered
or protected, but if we have an abscessing area or pyorrhea pocket one-
eighth of an inch deep around each tooth in the head how many square
inches of abscessing area do you suppose we have? Four square inches.
Now, what surgeon or physician would allow his patient to go for one
moment with that much suppurating surface from which infection can come,
and yet we pay no attention to it because it is in the mouth. Now, the large
part of infection seems to enter the system by means of the blood stream,
and the organisms pass through these large blood vessels into the smaller
ones and finally overcome the capillaries, and the blood has the property
of causing a coagulation so to speak, a grouping or clumping of the
bacteria, and that clumping makes it possible for them to block up these
little end arteries, and you will see that process taking place when we come
to the later pictures. We have some very interesting cases of this blocking
of the arteries. (Pictures were shown of stomach infection and skin
infection and so on.)

I presume no work of this decade is so valuable and significant as that
of Dr. E. C. Rosenow, formerly of Chicago, but now of the Mayo Institute.
He has shown when he has taken the germ from an appendix for example
and inocculated it into animals that the lesions produced in that animal
would in 68 per cent. of the cases be the appendix of the animal. That
means that organisms have a specific selective action for certain tissues. The
strain taken from the appendix selected the appendix in the animals, where
if the organism was taken from streptococcal cultures from other sources
than the appendix, only 5 per cent. had infections of the appendix. It is the
same way with the stomach ulcer, 65 per cent. had infection of the stomach
when it was taken from the stomach, and only 20 per cent. when it was
taken from miscellaneous infections, and it seems to follow on through in
the same way. What does that mean? He suggests it means this, if you
and I have an infection in our mouth that is selecting out our liver or our
appendix or our stomach and producing stomach ulcer, that germ may have
so definite and aggravated a form that if we place it on a drinking cup and
somebody else takes it off that drinking cup we may possibly transfer to
that person an infection of gall stones, an infection of peptic ulcer, or some
other infection of the body. That seems almost too far to take the possibili-
ties of this, and yet who knows but that may be true. The thing that
seems to be suggested to us is that we must be exceedingly careful to keep

our mouths just as clean as possible and prevent the possibility of carrying it to others. Dr. Rosenow has done probably the most important work that has ever been done with respect to mutations of organisms, and in this slide we see illustrations of his work. Some of the bacteriologists challenged his work and gave him a strain of pneumococcus and asked him to change it to streptococcus, and here we have an illustration. That means they are simply expressions of the same organism. Mutations are very unlikely to occur except in rare cases. Now, the medical men look in the patient's mouth to see whether or not he is suffering from a lead poisoning or mercury poisoning or phosphorus poisoning, simply because the most susceptible tissue of the entire body to poisons is the tissue surrounding the teeth, and that is probably the reason why pyorrhea is so prevalent. That susceptibility is shown so clearly in this case where some devitalizing paste was put into the tooth of this dog and with every precaution in sealing it into the tooth, using the cement and amalgam over the cement, yet the result of the amount of paste that passed through the apex or through the wall of the root and came back to the gingival border was enough not only to destroy the gingival border around those teeth in three days but to produce this necrotic area on each side of the tongue of the dog, showing the tremendous susceptibility of that tissue to the irritation of that drug. The next slide will show us some of the lesions at the apices of the root, but that is so large a subject we will not have time to dwell on it except to say that we of the dental profession should hesitate to use these things as the men of the medical profession and the surgeons hesitate to use bichloride of mercury in the abdominal cavity. A few years before that he used a rather strong solution of carbolic acid, but he does not use the strong solution of bichloride to-day, for he has found out that what kills the germs will kill the tissues, and he has found the thing he must do is to keep out of nature's way. We dental surgeons as a profession are still putting things into roots a dozen times too strong for the health of those tissues.

There is in the peridental tissue a network of cells running all the way from the gingival border to the apex of the root, and that chain or network seems to be a very important factor in the development of pyorrhea, for pyorrhea does not develop from a point around the tooth but develops continuously and progressively towards the apex of the root. Why this is so has never been solved, but it has been suggested partly by the finding of this network of epiphelial cells by Dr. Black, that it will be shown that that network is related to pyorrhea. We have in the mouth an organism that has caused a great deal of speculation in the last year or two, the ameba, but we do not believe it is important as being a factor in pyorrhea. We believe it is probably there because there is lots of food for it, which food is the breaking down lymphocytes and leukocytes. We do not believe, as I said, that it is to blame for pyorrhea.

Here is the picture of a young lady who has had a very sudden loss of her immunity. Suddenly her teeth are decaying very rapidly. The teeth were very sensitive. We have taken the debris from one of the cavities and put it on the microscopic slide, and you will note it is almost a pure culture. We then show a culture from that same patient's mouth showing organisms from other parts of the mouth, and you will notice an entirely different type and variety. On this slide we have an organism that has been blamed for pyorrhea and of being able to carry bacteria into tissue that is capable of infection. You will note how slowly it moves. (Shows various kinds of organisms.)

The next picture will show you these organisms which were taken from a blood system of a patient suffering from pyorrhea infection. We inoccu·lated a frog with a quantity of that organism, and it produced in the blood vessels of the frog the formations that I spoke of. You will see, first, the rhythmic motion of the lung of the frog. We cut a hole through the frog's back, so to speak, and then another hole through the anterior chest wall, and let the light go through the hole in the back and come out through the hole in the front, and we got this view of the circulation. We have, first, the rhythmic motion of the lung as it is stirred with the heart beat. You will notice the blood stream as it rushes through the veins and the arteries and the capillaries. We injected into the circulation two minims of a media carrying this organism, and the effect on the frog's blood was to cause what you might call clumps of bacteria blocking up the small end arteries, just as it happens to us in our bodies when we have an invasion of streptococci, or any other invasion of infection. The effect is a blocking of the end arteries and the formation of a clot. You will see the bacteria block up and block up, and then the pressure behind will break it up and it rushes away.

There was a time when you and I were one sole organism, very much like some of these organisms we have seen on the screen. We had many characteristics in common, so, as a matter of fact, they are very close cousins to us. Keep in mind three things now, for we will have to make these observations by inference: How do mutations occur by which new strains of bacteria develop in an abscess; second, how do these various forms of bacteria differ, and in what respects are they like ourselves, for, as a matter of fact, there was a time when each of us was a single germ cell, and at that time we were very, very much like these organisms we have been looking at, as you will see, and, thirdly, what are the conditions that determine the development of those organisms? The first of the pictures will show you the fertilizing process of certain forms of egg. I know of no operation in chemistry that is so rapid and so spectacular, and when you realize that practically all those processes are purely mechanical, it is wonderful. It is a process of physical chemistry. We will see how these bacteria produce the lesions they do and select the tissues they do without any conscious effort and without any influence except purely a matter of chemistry and physics. The first film will show the fertilizing process of a form of sea life. These organisms deposit their eggs into the water and they are fertilized in the water, and they behave almost like bacteria. See how quickly these little male atoms rush to that egg purely by a chemical process, and the first one that gets in is the only one that gets in, and as it does so it produces a chemical action on this membrane which prevents any other germ from getting in. This chemical process is so rapid that it takes place in a very small fraction of a second. As soon as the egg is fertilized, it divides into two, and presently into four, and then we have formations of eight. Here is an egg that did not fertilize, and you see the mass of germs that have been attracted purely by chemical attraction. Now, that process means that this nucleus of life has had carried into it the determiners of character and the determiners of resistance, and as it has been carried into it, it has been subject to modification of environment. Now, the thing I want to emphasize is, there is one condition under which an influence may take place, put there rapidly and rapidly modified, that is the determiner of the resistance of the body. Those are principally just when the membrane is forming in the early stages of development, and that may throw some light on why some people are subject to typhoid or inflammatory rheumatism, and so on. You will notice how these eggs separate or part as soon as the first germ enters, and that chemical process takes place, as I said, in a few seconds and is a physical operation that we can hardly conceive of, because of its rapidity. It is not difficult to modify that development process by the addition of very small quantities of chemicals, and very many people are susceptible to disease because at the time they were being fertilized as embryonic forms of life one of the parents, or both, was under the influence of alcohol, or the mother was suffering from the retention of some systemic poison—acid particularly, probably; and you will see some pictures of what was caused by the addition of a very small portion of alcohol, and how it is capable of making monstrosities, some with only one eye or with the eyes too close together, or, in some cases, serious head deformities and nervous deformities. The same deformities are produced in guinea pigs. In this case you can see the heart beat in this embryonic form of life. Here is one showing a head deformity on account of being treated when it was an egg with a very small percentage of alcohol. Many people have their resistance lowered because of influences that have come into their lives at the time that the determiners were being transferred through this very sensitive stage. In contrast to that, you see here a few cells of tissue taken from a frog's throat, which would be identical to those taken from the human throat. Here is a specimen showing two mouths, and if we cut the head off entirely and cut it up in sections, they will respond to food just exactly as if the rest of the body were there, show-ing it is an entirely mechanical process.   Here we have a young squid, and you will notice it has a sucking bottle.   Nature gives some of these organ-isms a quantity of food to sustain them for a time.   You can see him drink-ing out of his sucking bottle.   Here we have a pair of twins with their backs fastened together.   Here is a monstrosity simply because we added a little alcohol to the sea water in which it was developing.

In conclusion, I want to show you how mechanical they are when un-der an electric current.   They couldn't go in any other direction if they wanted to, and they turn in whichever direction the current is changed. When the current is changed too quickly, they simply oscillate.

I thank you very much for your most splendid attention.   (Applause.)

At the close of Dr. Price's address, H. B. Anderson, M.D., C.M., on behalf of the Academy of Medicine and the audience, moved a vote of thanks to the speaker for his excellent address and extraordinary illustrations. F. Arnold Clarkson, M.B., in a clever and witty speech, seconded the motion.

President's Address ·

A. J. McDONAGH, D.D.S., L.D.S., Toronto, Ont.

Read before Annual Meeting of Canadian Oral Prophylactic Association,
January, 1916.

Gentlemen,—Another year has gone around, a momentous year in the history of the world; the events which have taken place in the year just past have had a wonderful effect on every phase of human society, and we in our little society unfortunately have not escaped the far-reaching influences resulting from the world's greatest and most sanguinary struggle.

We have been hampered in more ways than one, and we have been deprived of the active co-operation of several of our best members. Doctors (now Capt.) Gow, Capt. Mallory and Capt. Hume have taken up the cause of their country, sacrificing themselves and their practice, and are now helping the poor soldiers who are fighting at Salonika. We wish them all success and hope they will soon return and be again happy, healthful participants in the work of this Society.

In the last year we have also lost three good friends by death—Dr. J. B. Willmott, the respected and worthy Dean of our College, was a friend of the Association from its inception, and Dr. Doherty, whose presence we were fortunate to have with us at our last annual meeting, and also Dr. Minns, who was just recently a member of our Association. The loss of friends such as these can never be repaired.

As I said in the beginning, business conditions in the last year have been very much disturbed; in fact, for a time we had difficulty in doing any business at all. Last year you were good enough to elect an Advertising Committee, which would act in conjunction with the Executive. That committee formulated an excellent scheme of advertising, got all the information necessary and the contracts all ready to sign, but just when we were on the point of signing the contracts and putting the fruits of their labors to the test we were confronted with the unfortunate condition that we could not get enough goods to supply the demand. Kent & Son, having got contracts from the Army to supply brushes to them, and having, of course, lost some of their employees, have not been able to supply us with our brushes.

Lyman Bros. reported to us that, although they had seven hundred gross of tubes on order in the Old Country, they could not get one to put up Hutax Paste, and consequently we could not get the paste, so that advertising to create more business was out of the question.

Just about that time we came in contact with a gentleman, Mr. Greatrix, who is with us here to-night, whose services were available and who was willing to promote the good of our enterprise and to manage the business for us. Through Mr. Greatrix' efforts principally, we have been able to induce Lyman Bros. to get a sufficient quantity of tubes from the United States to supply the immediate demand, and through him,- also, we have given a supplementary order to the Dupont people, of France, for one hundred gross of brushes, to be delivered as soon as possible; however, that will take time; in fact, it will be some time yet before the supply of our goods will be normal.

Notwithstanding all these drawbacks and the many factors which have militated against our progress during the past year, the sale of our brushes has increased by the substantial total of one hundred and thirteen gross, that of our paste and powder, forty gross.

In our Financial Secretary's report you will find there is one item left out, which could not be put in because the account for that item was not straightened up by the time of the annual report, and that is, at Christmas time, we donated powder and paste to about seventeen charitable institutions in the city, of a retail value of something over $175.00—the cost to us, of course, being less than that, as we got them at wholesale prices.

Our Educational Committee of last year and year before last has been working under difficulties, but our Secretary, Dr. Broughton, has been able to do a good deal of the work and has been able to assist the Educational Committee. The committee has been handicapped this year because Dr. Hume, who was a member, had to go to the military camp, and Dr. Grieve, the Secretary of the Committee, was forced to take up Dr. Hume's work at the College; besides, unfortunately, Dr. Grieve had the affliction of his wife dying, and through that, also, an extraordinary burden laid upon his shoulders.

This coming year your Executive hopes that the Educational Committee which you will appoint will undertake and do a great deal of the work which has devolved upon the Executive up to the present time; in fact, we hope to carry out the suggestion made by the Educational Committee that they meet at the same time and with the Executive.

It has been suggested that this Association provide a certain sum of money as a permanent endowment for research, and your Executive respectfully request that you express an opinion on that subject this evening. The Educational Committee will report the work done throughout the Dominion.

I want to thank the members of the Society for their loyal support in the past, and particularly the members of the Executive Committee, who have, as usual, thought no work of the Society a burden. I want, also, to thank the members of the other committees and the auditors for their services to the Association.

Secretary-Treasurer's Report

The annual meeting of the Canadian Oral Prophylactic Association was held January 20th, 1916, at the Walker House, Toronto. Owing to the fact that the programme arranged for our annual meeting—a lecture by Dr. Weston A. Price, on Blood Circulation, illustrated by Moving Pictures—would be of special interest to all the profession, it was decided to go on with the business part of the meeting, the reception of reports, etc., adjourn to Monday, February 14th, for the programme and to invite all the members of the Dental Profession of Toronto and vicinity to hear Dr. Price's lecture.

President's Report presented by Dr. A. J. McDonagh.

Educational Committee's Report presented by Dr. Geo. W. Grieve.

Financial Report presented by Dr. A. J. Broughton.

Receipts		$2,699.17
Expenditures—Charity and Educational		$ 646.29
Donations to:—		
Canadian Dental Association for the Army Service Com		
mittee		$106.28
Sick Children's Hospital		50.00
Army Dental Fund of the C.D.A.		100.00
Sunnyside Orphanage		`3.48
Toronto University Hospital Corps	$36.06	
McGill Hospital Corps	25.38	
Army Service Corps	52.35	
		——— 113.79
Lantern slides		13.80
Oral hygiene charts		70.00
Exhibit at O.D.A. convention		32.64
Printing		156.30
Expenditures of operating		1,225.02
Balance for 1916		2,453.97
Assets		3,943.47

Total gain over preceding year in revenue, $385.55.

Total gain over preceding year in tooth brush sales, 113 gross.

Total gain over preceding year in paste and powder sales, 40 gross.

Made in the USA
Middletown, DE
22 September 2021